Reverse Diabetes: Proven Methods for Safely Lowering Blood Sugar and Reversing Diabetes without Drugs, Including Free 28 Day Recipe Plan

Table of Contents

Introduction

Welcome to and thank you for choosing **Reverse Diabetes: Proven Methods for Safely Lowering Blood Sugar and Reversing Diabetes without Drugs, Including Free 28 Day Recipe Plan.** Diabetes is generally considered a blood sugar problem but in reality, blood sugar problems are the end result and not the underlying cause. There are many contributing factors to consider when discussing diabetes and the aim of this book is to simplify and clarify an illness that can sometimes be a terribly scary and lonely condition to deal with. The hopes are that **Reverse Diabetes: Proven Methods for Safely Lowering Blood Sugar and Reversing Diabetes without Drugs, Including Free 28 Day Recipe Plan** will act as a helpful guide and provide support to the reader alongside their medical team in achieving their goal of reversing diabetes.The term to reverse diabetes, within this book is defined as a significant long term stability and improvement in blood sugar levels and insulin sensitivity with regard to (but not exclusive to) type 2 diabetes in particular. For example, if a sufferer of type 2 diabetes were able to lower their HbA1c to below 42 mmol/mol (6%) without the use of medicated insulin has successfully reversed their diabetes and it is now in remission. When considering any lifestyle changes in the name of controlling/reversing diabetes the first thing to do is consult your GP and/or medical team and discuss the applicable risks. Failing to do so may complicate and exacerbate the existing illness(s) resulting in **Hyperglycaemia** and other life threatening conditions. First, we will cover the basics of diabetes, the most common diabetic conditions and a number of the factors that contribute to a diabetic diagnosis, followed by proven methods of management for reversing diabetes such as mind management and daily routine tips. The book finishes with a 28 day recipe plan full of delicious recipes that promote a healthy lifestyle. There are even a few extra recipes for delicious and healthy snacks to combat those mid-afternoon cravings.

As many as 1 in 3 of the adult population is shown to have prediabetes, a condition that pre-empts the onset of diabetes and so it's becoming ever more important that we act to reverse/control and prevent diabetic conditions through our actions before these pre-existing precursors develop into more serious conditions. But it's not all bad news; we all have the ability to manage and control our diabetes if we have the will to commit to dietary and lifestyle changes and the great thing is these changes will have a leveraging effect, improving many aspects of our lives at once. The results often include an overall healthier lifestyle with increased stamina and energy levels, improved circulation, healthy weight loss and a greater sense of control. Now, let's **Reverse Diabetes**.

What is Diabetes?

Diabetes is generally described as a disease which impairs the body's natural ability to either produce or respond to insulin, resulting in inflated levels of glucose in the blood. When healthy, our bodies produce insulin by way of the pancreas, which when released into the body acts to facilitate the movement of glucose into our cells, where it is then turned into energy. Insulin is an extremely important hormone without which we would all surely die. If our bodies are producing either inactive insulin or none at all, this can and probably will result in being diagnosed with one of many differing diabetic conditions. All of our cells use sugars (glucose) for energy; however, our bodies only require glucose in moderation. Too much glucose in the blood is highly detrimental and over time can seriously damage our kidneys, hearts and even our eyes. We will cover type 1 and type 2 diabetes in greater depth later on but in the meantime here's an analogy to make things a little clearer. If we imagine cells as locked boxes and insulin as the key that opens the boxes to allows the glucose to enter, we can describe type 1 diabetes in the following way:

- The body attacks the cells that produce insulin so there is no key and so the box stays locked.

And type 2:

- The key (insulin) is there but it does not fit the lock effectively and so the box stays locked.

In both of the aforementioned analogies the box stays locked; the glucose cannot enter the cells as required and therefore it builds up in the blood leading to hypoglycaemia.

Generally speaking, everyone is aware of types 1 and 2 and gestational diabetes as these are relatively well known, however, there are a number of other diabetic conditions that are less common and sometimes are misdiagnosed altogether. When successfully diagnosed type 1 diabetes sufferers and some type 2 sufferers will be prescribed either insulin pills or injections to ensure the body has enough insulin but even medicated insulin is not without its risks, raised insulin levels within the body can cause adverse effects such as:

- The retention of both water and salt resulting in raised blood pressure.

- Greater susceptibility to other diabetic conditions.

- A raised risk of atherosclerosis which may result in heart attack.

- Excess insulin may increase VLDL levels (Very Low Density Lipoprotein) and raises cholesterol.

What Causes Diabetes?

There is no single definitive factor that is known to cause diabetes but there are many factors that contribute to various diabetic conditions. The reason there is no single definitive cause for diabetes is due to the fact that there are numerous types of diabetes all with their own causes and precursors. Type 1 diabetes is caused by an autoimmune reaction that destroys the body's insulin producing cells whereas type 2 diabetes is usually caused by many factors working together culminating in what can best be described as an unhealthy lifestyle and poor diet as well as genetic precursors like family medical history and ancestry. There are some commonalities and triggers that affect the overwhelming majority of diabetic cases, especially the chronic cases, for example:

Type 1

- Genetic disposition.
- Viral infection.
- Ingestion of (unrelated to diabetes) toxins.
- Unrelated autoimmune reaction.

Type 2

- Age- over 40s.
- Sedentary lifestyle.
- Overweight or obese.

- Poor diet, binge eating, excess sugary snacks and refined carbohydrates.
- Ancestry.
- Medical history.

There are many more factors that can add to the potential risk factor and susceptibility to diabetes of all kinds:

- Cushing's syndrome may lead to diabetes as it causes excess levels of cortisol which in turn raises glucose levels. If the excess cortisol is not dealt with Cushing's syndrome will result in diabetes.
- Glucagonoma can cause the production of both glucagon and insulin to be unbalanced; if unchecked this may lead to hypoglycaemia and diabetes.
- Steroid induced diabetes.
- Pancreatitis may affect the body's natural ability to produce insulin, resulting in diabetic conditions.

Type 1

Type 1 diabetes is a disease that causes the body to attack the cells that create insulin and usually develops once around 90% of the insulin producing cells have been destroyed. Type 1 diabetes is classed as an autoimmune condition due to the body destroying insulin-producing cells, meaning that no insulin can be produced and it is this that leads to dangerously elevated glucose blood sugar levels and hypoglycaemia. Type 1 diabetes is a life-long condition that requires insulin to be medicated in either pill form or by injection to ensure the sufferer's blood sugar levels remain normal and within a safe range. Daily injections may seem a bit scary but insulin is a vital hormone, needed in the process of turning foods into energy. A lack of insulin can be life threatening and must be treated as such.

- 10%-15% of diabetes sufferers are diagnosed as suffering from **Type 1 Diabetes**.

The symptoms of type 1 diabetes can sometimes go unnoticed for a short period of time and at other times can have a sudden and rapid onset. The standard symptoms to be aware include but are not limited to the following:

- Irritability.
- Blurred vision.

- Weight loss or difficulty in gaining weight.
- Muscle loss.
- Prolonged and/or extreme thirst.
- Prolonged and/or extreme hunger.
- Fatigue and feeling tired all the time.
- A feeling of general weakness of the body.
- Urgent and frequent urination.
- Mood changes.
- Intimate itching.
- Skin irritation.
- Random and unexpected muscle cramps.
- Dizziness.

In addition to the symptoms mentioned above, the following are extreme symptoms, the sufferers of which require IMMEDIATE MEDICAL ATTENTION:

- Extremely high temperature.
- Stomach pains.
- Nausea and vomiting.
- Prolonged loss of appetite.
- Breath smells like chemicals, not unlike varnish.

Type 1 diabetes cannot be cured; however, at times the symptoms may disappear for up to a year only to reappear when the patient falls ill with a separate unconnected illness like a virus or the flu. As the body attacks the insulin producing cells, sufferers of type 1 diabetes become more and more dependent on insulin, lifestyle change may keep the need for medicated insulin to a minimum but make no mistake the process that destroyed 90% of the body's insulin producing cells does not stop at 90% and may eventually eradicate all of the body's insulin producing cells meaning the patient is completely reliant on outside sources of insulin. To successfully manage type 1 diabetes we must first keep up with prescribed insulin medications as well as taking up a healthy diet and exercise routine. This is true even if all the symptoms of diabetes seem to have gone away. It is important to keep taking insulin because this will help to maintain the remaining insulin producing cells. Failing to do so may eventually result in further diabetes related conditions like **Diabetic Ketoacidosis** which is usually associated with type 1 diabetes, however, type 2 sufferers may also be afflicted by this life threateningly dangerous complication which arises when the body all but runs out of insulin.

If you suspect that either you or anyone around you is affected by diabetic ketoacidosis it is important to seek IMMEDIATE MEDICAL ATTENTION as this complication can result in coma or even death when not acted upon at the earliest opportunity.

Type 2

Type 2 diabetes is the most common type of diabetes and occurs when the cells of the body that produce insulin either produce very low levels of insulin and/or the insulin produced by the cells is ineffective, this is generally known as insulin resistance. The insulin cannot properly unlock the cells and so glucose is allowed to build up and blood sugar levels rise. When we eat, the stomach breaks down food and converts it to glucose. The glucose is then allowed into the bloodstream. Insulin (created by the pancreas) is also released into the blood stream to facilitate the movement of glucose from the bloodstream to individual cells, however, in type 2 diabetes, the build-up of glucose stops the cells functioning properly. This build-up of glucose and resulting spike in blood sugar levels can result in the following complications:

- **Serious dehydration** happens when glucose levels are allowed to build up and it becomes too much for the kidneys to handle. This causes excess sugars to develop in the urine. These sugars draw water to them which results in a frequent and urgent need to urinate.
- **Nerve damage** and **narrowing of the arteries** can develop over time if raised glucose levels

are not properly managed which can result in heart attack and stroke.

- **Hyperosmolar hyperglycaemic non-ketotic syndrome**, otherwise known as **diabetic coma** is a continuation of serious dehydration and can arise if a sufferer of type 2 diabetes is unable to properly replace the fluids they have lost. Diabetic coma is an extremely serious and life threatening condition that can result in further complications later on.
- **Nephropathy** and other **kidneys diseases** can also develop if type 2 diabetes is not properly managed.

Typically, type 2 diabetes affects those over 40; however, those with a family background of Chinese, African-Caribbean, Middle Eastern or South Asian descent seem to be at risk of type 2 diabetes from around the age of 25. In recent times and in due to unhealthy diets and sedentary lifestyles type 2 diabetes has been seen to develop in younger people and even children across all ethnic groups.

The causes of type 2 diabetes also vary from type 1 as type 2 is generally caused by environmental factors such as lifestyle and diet and can be managed, symptoms reversed and prevented with planning and effort.

- 85%-90% of sufferers are diagnosed as suffering from Type 2 Diabetes.
- Most cases of Type 2 Diabetes are due to lifestyle and diet choices.
- Up to 58% of type 2 diabetes cases can be delayed and sometimes prevented altogether.

Sometimes sufferers of type 2 diabetes discover that the losing of any excess weight results in blood sugar levels returning to normal and the diabetic symptoms may disappear altogether. This does not mean that diabetes has disappeared, only that it is now in remission, likely due to a healthy diet and psychical activity and that their glucose level is probably still at a higher level on average than a healthy non-diabetic person. Type 2 diabetes takes a long time to develop and the body to takes a long time to get over its impaired glucose sensitivity, so do not be fooled into thinking less frequent symptoms means the disease is cured. When exercise routines are forgotten or our diets become lazy, we can quickly relapse into type 2 diabetes, this is especially true in times of stress.

Gestational Diabetes

Gestational diabetes mellitis (GDM) or Hypoglycaemia during pregnancy is a condition that only occurs during pregnancy; however, it can be caused by a pre-existing diabetic condition. If gestational diabetes is not properly managed, the risk of contracting type 2 diabetes after the pregnancy is greatly increased. Usually appearing in the latter stages of pregnancy, gestational diabetes is like other diabetic conditions in that it is indicative of blood sugar levels that are not properly regulated. This may be due to a general lack of insulin but can also be caused by the placenta releasing hormones that actually block the insulin.If you are planning to get pregnant and you have any concerns book an appointment with your local doctor who will alert you to any immediate issues and advise on the best course of action to take. If you have a family history of gestational diabetes let your doctor or midwife know at the earliest opportunity and they will be able to factor this into your pregnancy and birthing plan. If you are at significant risk of developing gestational diabetes your midwife or doctor may refer you to a specialist known as an endocrinologist who specialises in diabetes, if you face a lower risk you may be referred to a registered diabetes educator or even a dietitian all of which will be able to help you manage and maintain a healthy blood sugar level.

Who has the highest risk of developing gestational diabetes?

- Those who have previously had babies weighing greater than 10lbs (4.5k).
- Those with a BMI (Body Mass Index) greater than 30.
- History of gestational diabetes.
- Family background of Chinese, African-Caribbean, Middle Eastern or South Asian descent.
- Those with a poor diet and non-active lifestyle.

What are the symptoms to look out for?

- Increased or prolonged thirst as well as a dry mouth.
- Frequent urination.
- Lacking energy and/or feeling weak.
- Prolonged tiredness.

Suffering from the above symptoms can be normal for many pregnancies so don't worry too much if they arise but be sure to undergo a gestational diabetes test if the symptoms are severe or prolonged. If in any doubt contact your local GP, medical team or midwife.

When diagnosed with gestational diabetes frequent check-ups will be required in addition to the usual pre-natal checks to ensure blood sugar levels are consistent. Post pregnancy your doctor or referred specialist will continue to monitor your blood sugar levels for a further 6-8 weeks. It is common for gestational diabetes to fade away after the pregnancy but the extra checks are required to ensure that type 2 diabetes hasn't developed since the birth and if it has, that it is diagnosed as early as possible. When gestational diabetes goes untreated it can increase risks during birth as well as increasing the chances of the child contracting diabetes later on in life, for these reasons it is extremely important to diagnose gestational diabetes at the earliest possible opportunity.

Developing gestational diabetes can be especially troubling as it can directly affect the wellbeing of an unborn child but with a little bit of planning and a little extra care, there are ways to combat and stave off gestational diabetes. Completing a regular exercise routine will release a steady stream of endorphins which will lower stress levels as well as lowering the health risks to both mother and child. If you or someone close to you is affected by gestational diabetes please contact one of the many support groups out there who can properly help and advise those suffering both mentally and physically from the effects of gestational diabetes.

Macrosomia is a condition that arises through gestational diabetes that causes the child to be born with a larger than average body which can then lead to serious problems during the birth. Further to macrosomia. Gestational diabetes (especially if not diagnosed in the early stages) may affect pregnancy in the following ways:

- Could cause a **premature birth**.
- Could result in **Pre-eclampsia** which is a condition that causes high blood pressure and may lead to further complications.
- Could result in **Polyhydramnios** (excess amniotic fluid) and may lead to difficulties during labour.
- Abnormal development, congenital abnormalities affecting the nervous system and/or heart.
- **Jaundice.**
- **Respiratory Distress Syndrome.**
- **Diabetes in later life.**
- **Obesity.**
- **Stillbirth** (worst case scenario).

The above mentioned conditions are all exceptionally serious and should be treated as such as they have the potential to result in an early death. Here are some of the precursors and warning signs that my lead to gestational diabetes:

- Pre-existing diabetic conditions.
- Pre-existing glycosuria (sugar in the urine)
- Obesity.
- Previous sufferer of Polycystic Ovary Syndrome or PCOS.
- A family history of any diabetic conditions.
- Overweight before pregnancy
- Over 25 years old.

When it comes to gestational diabetes, prevention is the best form of treatment. The following will help to lower the risk of developing gestational diabetes both before and during pregnancy:

- Determine your risk factor.
- Up your fibre intake by 8g-10g per day.
- Up your protein intake.
- Make an effort to lose any excess weight either before or early on in the pregnancy.
- Keep active before and throughout pregnancy.
- Write out a pregnancy plan (but be flexible).

- Take an initial glucose challenge test followed up by a glucose tolerance test.
- Have a diabetes test every 3 months prior to and throughout the pregnancy.
- Follow any and all advice from your doctor, midwife or specialist.

Being diagnosed with gestational diabetes will mean making some changes to your lifestyle including but not limited to:

- Committing to an exercise routine.
- Monitoring your diet. Please see the 28 day recipe plan at the end of this book.
- Monitoring your blood sugar levels on a daily basis.
- More frequent visits with your doctor, midwife or specialist.
- Changes to your anticipated birth plan.

The long term effects of gestational diabetes could mean that you are at greater risk of developing gestational diabetes during future pregnancies as well as resulting in type 2 diabetes after the birth. If you have a history of gestational diabetes and are planning to get pregnant, request a diabetes test through your doctor prior to getting pregnant and if diagnosed with diabetes speak with your doctor about being referred to a diabetes pre-conception clinic that will be able to help manage your condition to allow for the safest pregnancy possible.

Preventing, Managing and Reversing Diabetes

Medicating diabetes (type 2 in particular) taking medicated insulin with addressing the real problem of insulin resistance is just a case of treating the symptoms. There's only one way to effectively reverse type 2 diabetes, by pushing it into remission and that's by dealing with the underlying cause, which ultimately is a resistance to insulin. To do this we must first cut out the carbohydrates and refined sugars that cause the body to produce insulin. If we constantly consume these types of foods and flood our systems with insulin the cells of the body become desensitised to the insulin and so diabetes can progress. By cutting these foods out we can stabilise our insulin production. Once we have stabilised our body's insulin production we can focus on insulin sensitivity. Insulin sensitivity can be increased through a steady exercise routine. Further to diet alone, techniques like intermittent fasting have been known to help lower and stabilise insulin levels. By taking our calories and carbohydrates at a set time in the day and fasting for the rest of the day we lower our insulin production and when this is carefully managed with light exercise results in increased insulin sensitivity and works particularly well with chronically and prolonged elevated insulin levels. In this section we will cover Mind Management, Daily Routine, Exercise, and Diet but further to these here are a few tips to get us started:

- Always sit at a table to eat. Sitting at the table to eat promotes good eating habits and stops mindless eating patterns that come with snacking on the move or on the sofa.
- Limit snacks should be kept to foods that are high in healthy fats like nuts, hummus and olives.
- Up your healthy fat intake, great sources of healthy fats include almonds, oily fish and avocado.
- Forget 5 day, make it 8-10 portions of colourful fruit and veg per day.
- Concentrate on quality; carb counting comes second to ensuring the carbs you consume are of the highest possible quality.
- Avoid added sugar anything like your life depended on it.
- One of the hardest tips to follow is to avoid all refined carbohydrates which include pasta, rice and breads (even whole grain).
- Eat quality proteins with as many meals as possible; this will maintain a feeling of fullness for longer lessening the need for snacks.

- Eat at set times every day, this helps to stabilise both insulin production and insulin sensitivity.

Mind Management

It's not easy to come to terms with lifelong conditions like diabetes, implementing the life changes that come with diabetes of all types can be challenging to say the least. The important thing is to not let the stress factor get to you as stress itself has an impact on blood sugar levels which makes stress especially harmful to those diagnosed with all types of diabetes. When suffering from stress our bodies release hormones like cortisol that give our cells access to energy stores of fats and glucose causing blood sugar levels to spike. Modern life is stressful, we live in a high pressure society with many factors contributing to our overall mental state and it is important that we recognise and manage these factors if we are to keep our stress levels to a minimum. Frustration and stress can also lead to depression which makes paying proper attention to diet and/or medication unlikely and can cause unnecessary risks. Regular stress will result in poor insulin sensitivity, unstable blood sugar levels and diabetes burnout. The term diabetes burnout refers to individuals who due to stress neglect their dietary needs or fail to regularly check their glucose levels. Sufferers from diabetes burnout are often disillusioned, disheartened and have submitted to diabetes believing their situation will never improve but this is not the case, change is constant and with a little work and self-confidence we can manage mental stress and be much healthier for it. Physical injuries, illnesses and general physical stresses also cause spikes in, and unstable blood sugar levels, therefore when required; rest and relaxation are pivotal in managing our overall stress levels and are an important part of preventing/managing/reversing diabetes. Practicing mindfulness, breathing techniques and practicing meditation are all known to work wonders when dealing with stressful situations. Taking as little as 10 minutes out every day to focus on meditation and breathing exercises lowers stress, cortisol levels and promotes normal blood levels.

Studies have shown that those with a high pressure working environment as well as a poor diet are 45% more likely of developing type 2 diabetes. Depression has also been known to raise the risk of contracting diabetes by around 17% and those who suffer from a diabetic condition are 29% more likely to also suffer from depression with the figure raising a high as 59% for those using insulin. Here are some techniques and tips for dealing with stress when diabetic:

Essentialism can at first be a tricky concept to grasp but what's important to understand is that practicing essentialism does not mean following any kind of structured time management programme. **Essentialism** can be best summed up as the art of neglecting everything that is unimportant. Through recognising what is important and acting from that alone we can ignore the infinite distractions that surround us and take stock of what's important and relax whilst doing so.

Essentialists adopt a doctrine that asserts that certain concepts, ideals, and skills be taught to everyone regardless of current level of education, background or ability. These skills and lessons range from and include (but are not limited to):

- Financial education
- Living environment
- Stress management and relaxation
- Accelerated learning
- Practical skills
- Self-development
- Daily routines

The 20%-80% rule is THE rule to live by,, and don't worry there are no maths involved. The 20%-80% rule otherwise known as the Pareto principle states that around 80% of effects are due to 20% of the causes, therefore the remaining 20% of effects are due to 80% of the causes. Pareto came to this conclusion when he realised that 80% of the money in Italy was being made by 20% of the population. This rule pretty much dictates that much of work we do is less than effective at the best of times. In reality, the ratio is usually much higher than 20%<80% sometimes as high as 5%<95%. The 20%-80% rule can be applied to almost every aspect of life, especially stress. 80% of our stress caused by people we know is caused by 20% of the people for example. When applied to our finances the 20%-80% rule can be life changing as too when applied to our relationships.
Further tips:

- When we **exercise** we work off not only excess fats and stress but as an added bonus our brains respond by releasing endorphins which in turn relaxes us further.

- **Avoid** drugs and other forms of **self-medication** like coffee and cigarettes.

- Make **sleep** a priority.

- **Accepted what you cannot change.**

- Keep **a positive outlook**; it's easy to look at the bad side of things in times of stress.
- **Planning ahead** is a sure way to lower future stress.
- **Set goals**, accomplishing set goals is great for stress relief and extremely productive.
- **Set alarms** to remind you of scheduled appointments, exercise regimes and you medication timetable (if you have one).
- Set and keep a regular **sleep schedule** by going to bed at the same time every night.

Daily routine

Sticking to a routine can be challenging, especially when making changes that range across practically every aspect of our lives and fitting diabetes into an already hectic life is no different. It takes discipline and heaps of willpower to begin with but an effective daily routine that includes a healthy diet, work schedule, exercise and plenty of relaxation completely reinvigorates our lives. Be dedicated but not overly serious, don't stress yourself out with the minutia just create a routine that works for you, stick to it and it and in a week or two the flow will kick in and you'll never look back. Remember to enjoy yourself, don't forget to laugh, it relaxes us and bolsters the immune system. Developing and sticking to our daily routines acts to empower us and provides a sense of regularity and control which in turn will promote stabilised blood sugar levels over extended periods of time. Ultimately our daily routines must revolve around controlling our conditions before they can progress further. If left untreated diabetic conditions result in kidney failure, heart disease and strokes to name but a few and so it is crucial that we take the necessary steps to stop it in its tracks and if possible put it into remission. The lighter side of things is that the day to day management of diabetes is quite simple if we keep four main

points in mind:
- **Monitoring blood sugar levels**
- **Diabetic diet**
- **Exercise**
- **Relaxation**

A few important things to remember:
- Check glucose levels first thing in the morning.
- Eat a balanced breakfast.
- Check glucose levels at midday.
- Eat a balanced lunch.
- Take a 20 minute walk after eating lunch.
- If hungry in the mid-afternoon snack on some fruit or almonds.
- Eat a balanced dinner.
- 20 minutes light exercise or a 30 minute walk.
- Check glucose levels before going to bed.

Exercise

We all need to exercise, non-sufferers and sufferers of diabetes alike, it should go without saying, but unfortunately in modern society our lives are becoming more and more sedentary leaving most of us either desk-bound, sat in a car seat or lounging on the sofa the majority of the time. Regular exercise is a crucial component for a full and healthy life and this goes double for those living with diabetes, let alone those who wish to push diabetic their conditions into remission.

When we exercise and our muscles contract hormones are released that allow our cells to absorb glucose completely independent of insulin, this alone makes exercise one of the best things we can do to combat diabetes. Physical activities affect everyone differently, familiarising yourself with how your body reacts to different levels of exercise will allow you to design a diet and exercise plan that complement each other perfectly. If hypoglycaemia interrupts your exercise routine on a regular basis try snacking 30 minutes prior to exercising, it the hypoglycaemia persists contact your doctor to discuss making adjustments to your diabetes treatment plan and medication.

Some of us may find exercise more difficult than others, especially affected my fatigue but start simple, go slow and always consult your doctor beforehand and consider visiting your optician for a check-up. Start with a gentle walk every day before progressing to jogging; consider joining a cycling or swimming club and for the more daring among us hiking and mountain climbing are extremely rewarding. Aerobic exercise has been known to lower blood sugar levels, strengthen the heart, build stamina and improve insulin sensitivity resulting in lower diabetic risks and overall greater health. Strength training and a low fat diet is great for muscle growth but is also thought to be especially helpful to those with diabetes. Moderate aerobic exercise is particularly helpful to those suffering from type 1 diabetes as it not only improves sensitivity to insulin but also lowers both cholesterol and body fat. The American Diabetes Association recommends a minimum of 2½ hours (150 minutes) of moderate aerobic exercise or at least 1½ hours (90 minutes) or intense physical exercise per week. There's no need to exercise every day, exercise no more than two consecutive days to avoid strains and other injuries. Sufferers of diabetes are more susceptible to heart disease and so must consult their doctor or medical teams before taking on anything strenuous. High impact workouts are at first to be avoided by

those whose diabetes is not yet under control as
the impact from such exercises can weaken
already damaged blood vessels within the eyes
of sufferers of retinopathy (a commonplace
diabetic condition) and can also have a
detrimental effect on the blood vessels within
the feet. To exercise safely diabetics must take
the necessary precautions and be aware of
certain facts if we are to exercise safely and
effectively:

- Always keep 15g-20g of fast acting carbs 'to hand' at all times in case you experience hypoglycaemia whilst exercising.
- Eat within 90 minutes of exercising.
- Glucose levels can spike and drop massively during exercise and so should be measured before, during and after a workout.
- Drink plenty of fluids prior to exercising.
- Go at a steady pace.
- Do not exercise for extended periods or over strenuously.
- The insulin dependent exerciser may require lower insulin doses or to eat more carbohydrates, prior to exercise. Although, they may have need of an extra dose of insulin.
- Take a rest day if glucose levels are above 300mg/dl or lower than 100mg/dl.

Diet

It's not only about sugars we must also be vigilant when dealing with fats (especially Trans fats) as well as our sodium intake (salts). Like most things in life, it's not what you do that counts but how you do it and properly implementing new eating habits is harder than it seems. Carbohydrates have a huge impact on our glucose levels are one of the main nutrients we find throughout almost all of our foods and drinks includes not just sugars but fibre and starches also. Concentrating on complex carbohydrates is the best place to start. Complex carbohydrates break down slower and therefore release sugars at a lower rate making them easier for the body to manage. Whole grains, beans lots of starchy vegetables and fruits are essential. Some fruits are better than others such as:

- Apples are great for vitamins
- Apricots for fibre
- Blueberries and grapes for antioxidants
- Cherries fight inflammation
- Oranges for vitamin C
- Pears are full of fibre and vitamin K
- Peaches for potassium

It's the simple carbohydrates that we want to avoid, as well as those sweet sugar rushes we all crave but don't worry too much, after a few weeks these cravings do diminish and will eventually disappear. The most important thing we can do by way of diet if we are to manage diabetes is to eliminate the nasty sugars altogether, a few of the worst offenders are:

- Sweets, chocolate (all candy).
- Fizzy drinks.
- Juices and cordials from concentrate.
- Non whole grain baked goods.
- Processed meats.
- Fast food.
- Granulated sugar
- Coffee
- Crisps/Chips
- Nachos
- Deep fried foods
- Fruit juice drinks
- Biscuits, cakes and cookies
- Fried chicken
- Pizza
- Milkshakes
- Jams/Jelly
- Energy drinks
- Flavoured water

- White bread
- Bananas

The dietary advice for type 1 diabetes varies greatly but the central factor to be aware of in knowing what foods cause the greatest spike in your glucose levels, eliminating these troublesome sugars and replacing them with complex carbohydrates. This book does not recommend that anyone stop taking the insulin prescribed to them. Always consult your doctor or diabetes specialist before making any changes in the amount of insulin you are taking. Type 1 sufferers must learn to balance the correct complex carbohydrates with their medicated insulin, which may seem complicated but there are a number of resources available to help us count those carbs from websites and online courses to books and dietitians. Carb counting is a process that takes time and effort to master and will require considerable learning alongside the constant monitoring of our blood sugar levels but the payoff I well worth it. Getting to grips with carb counting will provide a greater feeling of control over diabetes which in turn provides the makings of a full and free life not weighed down by diabetes. If you are considering carb counting consult your doctor and/or diabetes specialist and with their support create a structured diet plan that can be measured and monitored. There are thousands of people out there who are living their lives to the fullest through mastering the art of carb counting and carefully balancing their food intake with their medicated insulin. When we get really good at carb counting we will be able to predict our blood sugar levels and the effects specific foods will have on us including time frame and overall impact on our glucose levels. Over time knowing exactly how specific foods and ingredients affect our systems gives us flexibility at meal times meaning we have greater control over when we eat, how much we eat and what carbs we eat. It is important to be aware of the fact that lowering your intake of carbohydrates will require a reduction in any medicated insulin and that a failure to do both correctly and safely could result in hypoglycaemia. **Always consult your medical team prior to any dietary changes.**

Type 2 diabetes and/or gestational diabetes is not something we can simply eat our way out of. To manage, prevent or reverse these conditions we must integrate the proper diet with a number of other controlled methods in order to achieve the best results and carb counting is again the best place to start. But with that being said it is possible to put type 2 and gestational diabetes into remission with Low-carb, low-calorie, often Mediterranean style diet. Low-fat diets have been tested alongside Mediterranean diets and both do have a positive effect on type 2 diabetes, however, the Mediterranean diet has proven to have a greater impact over a shorter time, putting type 2 diabetes into remission in as little as three months when taken alongside proper exercise and other lifestyle changes. Lean meats, skinless grilled chicken and oily fish are great sources of protein which the body breaks down at much slower rate than carbohydrates and so has a lower impact on blood sugar levels. If you must have bread, switch to whole grain, and with rice switch to brown but if you are truly serious about reversing diabetes it is advised to cut out both completely.

Carb Counting Tips:

- **Work with your doctor**, you're not alone.
- Don't be afraid of asking for help.
- The hardest part is starting.
- Keep an eye on portion sizes.
- Use an App.
- Read the nutritional values on food.
- Be accurate in your counting.
- Keep a food diary.
- Plan your meals ahead of time.
- Plan for long trips.
- Use your common sense.
- Eat homemade meals.
- NO TAKEAWAYS OR FAST FOOD.

- Learn the language, for example, low in fat usually means high in sugars.
- Monitor blood sugar levels regularly.

28 Day Recipe Plan

Low calorie diets consisting of mostly low-carb vegetables such as broccoli have been known to reverse type 2 diabetes. A 90 gram serving of broccoli will contain up to 4 grams of easily digestible carbohydrates as well as at least 2 grams of fibre and high amounts of vitamins C and K. It is well known that broccoli has inflammation fighting properties, reduces insulin resistance and can also defend against numerous cancers including prostate cancer. Asparagus is also a fantastic food for preventing and combatting diabetes and even acts to protect and promote healthy brain function and growth. A single portion of asparagus will contain around 8 grams of carbohydrates 4 of which are fibre. Just like broccoli, tests with asparagus have proven that asparagus may prevent growth in certain cancers as well as lowering anxiety. It's not just the greens, summer squash and zucchini carry high levels of vitamin C and are low in carbs, winter squash has more carbohydrates than the summer and zucchini varieties but is still effective when part of a healthy diabetes reversing diet. Mushrooms have an average of only 2 grams of carbohydrates per serving one of which is fibre. Being high in antioxidants and having strong anti-inflammatory qualities as well as being as adaptable as they are delicious makes mushrooms an excellent addition to any diabetes preventing/reversing diet. Creating and sticking to a diabetic diet or healthy eating plan can at times feel difficult; however, it is essential if we are to manage our blood sugar levels. Monitoring our carbohydrate intake, swapping out ingredients and following healthy meal plans are ways in which we can combat and begin to manage diabetes. Once diagnosed with any kind of diabetes it is not uncommon to be referred to a specialist or dietitian who can properly advise upon and recommend the types of foods we should be eating and when. The recipe plan below is based on three meals per day at set times. This will help to the body to make effective use the insulin it produces or is being medicated. We can all improve our eating habits from portion control to the time of day that we choose to eat and there are registered dietitians who can help you to create full diet plans specifically tailored to both the individual and their diagnosis, however, for those of us creating our own diet plans or for anyone looking for a bit of inspiration in the kitchen below is your **28 Day Recipe Plan**. If there is ever any doubt surrounding a specific ingredient try checking its GI (Glycaemic Index) online at www.glycemicindex.com. The Glycaemic Index measures foods by how fast they raise the body's blood sugar levels. Foods that score below 50 have a low glycaemic index whilst foods that score over 70 should generally be avoided. The recipes below were designed to promote healthy living, help to prevent and manage diabetes and protect against heart problems and inflammation related conditions. Generally, it is considered a good idea to completely cut out all refined carbohydrates that come in the form of pasta, rice and breads, however, in a small number of recipes that follow contain brown rice or bread as an optional side. This was done not only to add a little diversity to the proposed recipe guide but to also take into account that everyone is different and that some people may have been advised to consume small amounts of carbs in the form of brown rice or a slice or two of wholemeal bread once or twice a week. Please enjoy.

Day 1
Breakfast
Cucumber, Ginger and Pineapple Breakfast Smoothie
Ingredients
1 cup of pineapple chunks
½ cucumber, peeled and roughly chopped
½ cup of ice cubes
½ teaspoon of freshly grated ginger
¼ teaspoon of cinnamon
¼ teaspoon of turmeric
5-8 mint leaves
½ cup of green tea,, cooled
½ cup of water
Method
1. Place all of the ingredients into a food processor or blender and blend until smooth.

Serving your Mango, Ginger and Pineapple Smoothie
Serve immediately in a tall glass with a sprinkling of chia seeds.

Lunch
Mediterranean Tuna Salad
Ingredients
2 tins of tuna in spring water (4 servings)
¼ cup mixed olives
¼ cup finely chopped red onion
¼ cup chopped oven roasted red pepper
3 cherry tomatoes, chopped
150g spinach leaves
1 handful chopped lettuce
¼ handful chopped basil leaves
¼ cup sliced cucumber
Salt and ground black pepper to taste
Mayonnaise (optional)
Method
1. Using a large bowl mix the tuna, lettuce, cucumbers, tomatoes, olives, onion, red pepper, basil and a little salt and pepper to taste.
2. At this point, it is optional to add 2-3 tablespoons of mayonnaise.

Serving your Mediterranean Tuna Salad
Serve chilled atop a bed of mixed green leaves.

Dinner
Dry Rub Steak
Ingredients
2 large sirloin or fillet steaks
2 cloves of garlic, grated
1 inch ginger, grated
½ teaspoon cumin
½ teaspoon coriander
½ teaspoon cinnamon
½ teaspoon allspice
Salt to taste
Method
1. Mix the garlic, ginger, cumin, coriander, cinnamon, allspice and a little salt to taste in a bowl.
2. Coat the steaks in the mix evenly on both sides and refrigerate for at least 30 minutes.
3. Grill the steaks for 4-6 minutes on each side depending on individual taste.
4. Once cooked rest the steak for 2 minutes.

Serving your Dry Rub Spiced Steak
Serve hot with mixed green leaves.

Day 2
Breakfast
Smoked Salmon and Potato Rosti
Ingredients
1 large russet or Maris Piper potato
1 tablespoon of butter
110g soft goat cheese chopped into small cubes
Thinly sliced smoked salmon
1 clove of garlic, grated
2 teaspoons of freshly grated ginger
Zest of ½ a lemon
¼ red onion, finely chopped
½ a tomato, chopped
1 small handful of chopped spinach leaves
Method- Rosti

1. Peel the potato and grate into a bowl.

2. Rinse the grated potato with water to remove any excess starch and then squeeze the potato hard in your hands to remove any liquids.

3. Season the potato with salt and ground black pepper.

4. Place the butter in a frying pan or skillet and melt over a medium heat.

5. Whilst the butter melts, shape the potato mix into burger shapes.

6. Place the potato in the frying pan or skillet and cook for 16-18 minutes turning midway.

7. Once cooked place your potato rosti to one
    side.

Method- Topping
1. In a bowl, mix the goat cheese, spinach
    leaves, onion, tomato, garlic, lemon zest,
    ginger and a little salt and ground black
    pepper to taste.

Serving your Smoked Salmon and Potato Rosti
Spoon some of the topping mix on to the rostie
and place a couple of layers of smoked salmon
on top, serve warm.

Lunch
Citrus, Avocado and Green Leaf Salad
Ingredients
½ pink grapefruit peeled, sliced and segmented
1 Valencia orange peeled, sliced and segmented
1 tablespoon of finely grated or minced shallots
1 avocado, sliced
Mixed fresh salad greens
1 handful of spinach leaves
½ teaspoon of Dijon mustard
2 tablespoons of red wine vinegar
2 tablespoons olive oil
¼ cup sliced almonds
Salt and ground black pepper to taste
Method

1. In a bowl, whisk together the Dijon mustard, olive oil, shallots and red wine vinegar with a little salt and ground black pepper to taste.
2. Mix the pink grapefruit, oranges, avocado, spinach and green leaves in a bowl.

Serving your Citrus, Avocado and Green Leaf Salad
Toss the vinaigrette with the salad and serve.

Dinner
Garlic, Chili and Ginger Cod Loin with Green Leaves
Ingredients
2-4 cod loin fillets
3 cloves of garlic finely chopped
1 inch piece of ginger, grated
½ teaspoon of dried chili flakes
1 tablespoon of lemon juice
2 tablespoons of olive oil
Salt and ground black pepper to taste
Mixed green leaves
1 tomato, sliced
1 carrot, peeled and cut julienne
Method
1. Mix all of the ingredients and fully coat the cod loins ensuring they are evenly covered.
2. Heat some oil in a pan.
3. In a bowl toss the mixed green leaves, sliced tomato and carrot into a bowl.
4. Place the cod loins skin down in the pan, along with any remaining marinade and cook for 2-3 minutes or until the skin is crisp.
5. Gently turn the cod loins and cook for a further 2-3 minutes.

Serving your Garlic, Chili and Ginger Cod Loin with Green Leaves
Serve your cod loins hot atop a bed of salad.

Day 3
Breakfast
Salmon and Avocado on Toast
Ingredients
Bread (gluten free), toasted (optional)
1 avocado, sliced
1 packet of smoked salmon
¼ cup finely chopped radish sprouts
Salt and ground black pepper
Lemon juice
Method
1.   Top the toast with salmon and radish sprouts.

Serving your Salmon and Avocado on Toast
Serve with a little salt and ground black pepper along with a dash of lemon juice.

Lunch
Light Spice Butternut Squash and Lentil Stew
Ingredients
3 cups of butternut squash chopped and cooked
½ cup lentils
½ cup red lentils
1 cup of carrots, chopped
1 red onion, chopped
½ cup of broccoli, chopped
2 cloves of garlic, finely chopped
½ inch piece of fresh ginger, grated
800ml vegetable stock
½ teaspoon of turmeric
½ teaspoon of medium curry powder
1 tablespoon of olive oil
Salt and ground black pepper to taste
Method- Butternut squash
1. Chop the butternut squash and mix it in a bowl with a little olive oil, salt and pepper.
2. Place the butternut squash on a baking and into the oven at 190°F, cook for 20 minutes.

Method- Light Spice Butternut Squash and Lentil Stew
1. Heat the olive oil in a large cooking pot over a medium-high heat.
2. Add the onions to the pot and cook for 3 minutes.
3. Add the garlic and ginger to the pot and cook for a further 2 minutes.

4. Stir in the carrots, lentils, curry powder, turmeric, vegetable stock and bring to the boil, then reduce the heat and cook for 10-12 minutes.

5. Add the broccoli, butternut squash and a little salt and pepper to taste to the stew and cook for a further 10 minutes.

Serving your Light Spice Butternut Squash and Lentil Stew

Serve in serving bowls (4 servings) with a sprinkling of grated cheese.

Dinner
Garlic, Chili and Ginger Cod Loin with Green Leaves
Ingredients
2-4 cod loin fillets
3 cloves of garlic finely chopped
1 inch piece of ginger, grated
½ teaspoon of dried chili flakes
1 tablespoon of lemon juice
2 tablespoons of olive oil
Salt and ground black pepper to taste
Mixed green leaves
1 tomato, sliced
1 carrot, peeled and cut julienne
Method
1. Mix all of the ingredients and fully coat the cod loins ensuring they are evenly covered.
2. Heat some oil in a pan.
3. In a bowl toss the mixed green leaves, sliced tomato and carrot into a bowl.
4. Place the cod loins skin down in the pan, along with any remaining marinade and cook for 2-3 minutes or until the skin is crisp.
5. Gently turn the cod loins and cook for a further 2-3 minutes.

Serving your Garlic, Chili and Ginger Cod Loin with Green Leaves
Serve your cod loins hot atop a bed of salad.

Day 4
Breakfast
Smoked Salmon and Runny Egg on Toast
Ingredients
1 pack of smoked salmon
Thick cut gluten free bread
2 eggs per person
Salt and ground pepper to taste
1 tablespoon of butter
Method
1. Heat the butter in a non-stick frying pan or skillet over a medium-high heat.
2. Whilst the butter is melting place the bread under the grill, cook for3-4 minutes (or until toasted) turning midway.
3. Break the eggs and gently slide them into the pan, lower the heat to medium-low and cook until the whites become stiff and the yolk thickens.
4. Remove the salmon from the pack season with a little salt and ground pepper to taste.

Serving your Smoked Salmon and Runny Egg on Toast
Serve immediately, place the salmon on toast and place an egg on top.

Lunch
Beetroot Salad
Ingredients
1 ½ beetroot, grated or chopped julienne
1 carrot, grated or chopped julienne
1 pear, diced
1 apple, diced
1 clove garlic, grated or minced
1 cup mixed green leaves
1 tablespoon almonds
1 tablespoon hemp oil
Method

1. In a large mixing bowl mix together the beetroot, carrot, pear, apple, garlic, almonds and hemp oil.

Serving your Beetroot Salad
Serve immediately atop a bed of mixed green leaves.

Dinner
Ginger Beef and Broccoli Stir-Fry
Ingredients
500g sirloin beef steak cut into thin slices
2 cups of broccoli florets
1 cup of green beans, chopped
1 onion, chopped
1 medium sized carrot, peeled and sliced
julienne
1 cup of kale leaves, washed and chopped
2 garlic cloves, finely chopped
1 red pepper, sliced
1 teaspoon of turmeric
½ inch piece of fresh ginger, grated
2 tablespoons of wheat free tamari
1 tablespoon of fresh lemon juice
½ teaspoon of salt
½ teaspoon of ground black pepper
1 tablespoon of apple cider vinegar
1 ½ tablespoons of coconut oil
Method
1. Warm a frying pan over a medium-high heat, toss in and melt the coconut oil.

2. Add the garlic, red pepper, ginger and onion to the pan. Cook for 5-6 minutes.

3. Stir the beef slices into the pan and cook for a further 5-6 minutes.

4. Add the Turmeric, lemon juice, salt, pepper, carrot, kale leaves, broccoli, green beans and apple cider vinegar to the pan.

5. Stir well and cook over a medium heat for 13-
    15 minutes.

Serving your Ginger Beef and Broccoli Stir-Fry
Serve with brown rice and green leaf salad.

Day 5
Breakfast
Green Detox Smoothie
Ingredients (4 servings)
4 golden delicious apples, cored
2 pears, cored
2 cucumbers
1 cup of spinach
1 cup kale
½ a lemon
½ a lime
4 sticks of celery
1 teaspoon grated ginger root
Ground black pepper to taste (optional)
½ cup ice
Method
1. Blend or juice all of the ingredients.

Serving your Green Detox
Serve immediately.

Lunch
Zahtar Salmon with Citrus and Green leaf Salad
Ingredients
2 salmon fillets
1 ½ teaspoons of Zaatar spice
1 clove of garlic finely chopped
1 teaspoon of dried coriander
1 tablespoon of lemon juice
Salt and ground black pepper to taste
Olive oil
Mixed green leaves
1 tomato, sliced
1 carrot, peeled and cut julienne
Vinaigrette of choice
Method
1. Mix the zaatar, coriander, lemon juice, garlic, 1 tablespoon of olive oil and a little salt and ground black pepper to taste in a bowl.
2. Place the salmon fillets in the mix, coat thoroughly, cover and place in the fridge for at least 30 minutes.
3. Warm a little oil in a pan over a medium heat.
4. Gently place the salmon fillets in the pan skin side down, pour any remaining marinade mix over the salmon and cook for 4-6minutes, carefully turning midway.
5. Toss together the mixed green leaves, sliced tomato, carrot slices and some salt and

pepper to taste and a little of your chosen vinaigrette.

Serving your Zaatar Salmon with Citrus and Green leaf Salad

Serve hot atop a bed of salad.

Dinner
Garlic and Mushroom Steak
Ingredients
2 large sirloin or fillet steaks
2 cloves of garlic, grated
1 cup button mushrooms, sliced
Salt and ground black pepper to taste
Olive oil
Method
1. Heat a frying pan or skillet over a medium-high heat and throw in the garlic and mushrooms a long with a drizzle of olive oil.
2. Season the steak with salt and pepper to taste, place the steaks into the frying pan or skillet and cook for 4-6 minutes each side depending on individual taste.
3. Once cooked allow the steak to rest for a few minutes before serving.

Serving your Garlic and Mushroom Steak
Serve hot alongside mixed green leaves.

Day 6
Breakfast
Smoked Salmon and Runny Egg on Toast
Ingredients
1 pack of smoked salmon
Thick cut gluten free bred
2 eggs per person
Salt and ground pepper to taste
1 tablespoon of butter
Method
1. Heat the butter in a non-stick frying pan or skillet over a medium-high heat.
2. Whilst the butter is melting place the bread under the grill, cook for3-4 minutes (or until toasted) turning midway.
3. Break the eggs and gently slide them into the pan, lower the heat to medium-low and cook until the whites become stiff and the yolk thickens.
4. Remove the salmon from the pack season with a little salt and ground pepper to taste.

Serving your Smoked Salmon and Runny Egg on Toast
Serve immediately, place the salmon on toast and place an egg on top.

Lunch
5 Minute Salad
Ingredients
4 cups lettuce
½ a cucumber
2 cups spinach
2 tomatoes, chopped
¼ cup black olives
1 cup grated carrot
½ cup chopped red onion
Method
1. Toss all of the vegetables in a bowl, drizzle a little olive oil and a little salt and pepper.

Serving your 5 Minute Salad
Serve immediately, alone or with literally anything.

Dinner
Lemon and Herb Cod
Ingredients
2-4 cod loin fillets
1 small handful of chopped basil leaves
1 ½ teaspoons of Italian mixed herbs
¼ cup chopped parsley
1 tablespoon of lemon juice
1 tablespoon of lime juice
2 tablespoons of olive oil
Salt and ground black pepper to taste
Method
Mix together the basil, Italian mixed herbs,
lemon juice, lime juice, chopped parsley, olive
oil and a little salt and pepper to taste.
Coat the cod loins in the mix, cover and
refrigerate for at least 30 minutes.
Heat some olive oil in a pan over a medium heat.
Place the cod loins into the pan, pour over any
remaining marinade and cook for 4-6 minutes,
turning midway.
Serving Lemon and Herb Cod
Serve with rice, spoon the juices from the pan
over the cod and rice.

Day 7
Breakfast
Smoked Salmon and Potato Rosti (recipe above).
Lunch
The Ultimate Veggie Burger
Ingredients
1 large sweet potato
½ cup red onion, finely chopped
2 cloves of garlic, grated
1/2 cup quinoa
¼ cup multi-purpose gluten free flour
½ cup black beans
¼ cup kidney beans
½ teaspoon cumin
¼ teaspoon paprika
2 teaspoons Cajun spice
Olive oil
½ cup watercress
1 cup lettuce
Salt and ground black pepper to taste
Method

1. Cook the quinoa as per the instructions on the pack.
2. Roast the sweet potato for 30 minutes (or until soft) in a pre-heated oven at 400°F/200°C (gas mark 6).
3. Allow the sweet potato to cool, remove the skin, place in a food processor alongside the garlic, red onions, paprika, Cajun spice,

cumin, kidney beans, black beans and salt and pepper to taste. Blend until almost smooth.

4. In a large bowl, mix together the sweet potato mix and quinoa along with a little flour (just enough so that burger shapes can be formed.

5. Divide the mix into 6-8 burger or patty shapes and refrigerate for 30 minutes.

6. Heat some olive oil in a frying pan or skillet and cook the burger for 5-6 minutes on either side or until they begin to brown.

Serving your Ultimate Veggie Burgers
Serve topped with lettuce and cress inside gluten free burger buns.

Dinner
Pan Seared Salmon and Mushrooms
Ingredients
2-4 skinless/deboned salmon fillets
1 cup sliced shitake mushrooms
½ tablespoon lemon juice
½ tablespoon lime juice
½ teaspoon medium-heat chili flakes
1 tablespoon black pepper
Salt to taste
½ tablespoon chopped chives
½ tablespoon parsley
Olive oil
Method
1. Heat 1 tablespoon of olive oil in a large frying pan or skillet on a medium heat.
2. Add the mushrooms to the pan along with the chili flakes and cook for 3 minutes.
3. Coat the top side of the salmon with black pepper, place into the frying pan and cook for 3 minutes before carefully turning and cooking for a further 2 minutes.
4. Remove the salmon from the frying pan and pour over the lemon and lime juices.

Serving your Pan Seared Salmon and Mushrooms
Garnish with chives and parsley, serve hot with brown quinoa.

Day 8
Breakfast
Spinach Bruschetta
Ingredients
Bruschetta
1 cup of spinach
½ red onion, minced
1 clove of garlic
Olive oil
½ cup Greek yoghurt
1 tablespoon fresh mint
Salt and ground black pepper to taste
¼ cup chopped walnuts
Method
1. Drizzle some olive oil over the bruschetta and place it in the oven for 5 minutes.
2. Whilst the bruschetta is toasting, boil the spinach for 3-5 minutes before draining off.
3. Heat some olive oil in a pan and sauté the onions and garlic for 3 minutes.
4. Mix the spinach, onions, garlic, yoghurt, walnuts and mint in a bowl.

Serving your Spinach Bruschetta
Serve the toasted bruschetta topped with the spinach mix.

Lunch
Thai Steamed Trout
Ingredients
2-4 trout deboned fillets
2 cloves of garlic, grated
½ inch piece of ginger, grated
¼ teaspoon medium-heat chili flakes
1 ½ teaspoon mixed Thai spice
1 teaspoon lemon juice
1 tablespoon soy sauce
1 tablespoon sesame oil
Salt and ground black pepper to taste
Method
1. In a bowl mix together the sesame oil, soy sauce, lemon juice, garlic, ginger, chili flakes, Thai spice and a little salt and pepper to taste.
2. Place the trout in the marinade, ensuring the fillets are fully coated and refrigerate for at least 2 hours.
3. Make a bed from tin foil, place the trout fillets inside and pour over the marinade.
4. Wrap the foil over, covering the trout and place in a pre-heated oven at 400°F/200°C (gas mark 6) for 15-18 minutes.

Serving your Thai Steamed Trout
Serve immediately with baked potato and mixed green leaves.

Dinner
Spiced Hamburgers
Ingredients
450g ground beef
2 cloves of garlic, grated
¼ teaspoon turmeric
½ red onion, finely chopped
1 teaspoon allspice
Lettuce
1 tomato
Salt and ground black pepper to taste
Olive oil
Method
1. Place the onion on a parchment lined baking tray, drizzle with olive oil and cook in a pre-heated oven on a medium heat for 6-8 minutes or until browning.
2. Mix the garlic, turmeric, onions, allspice and ground beef in a large bowl.
3. Using your hands form the beef mix into 4-6 burgers and refrigerate for 30 minutes.
4. Place the burgers under the grill for 15-18minutes turning regularly.

Serving your Spiced Hamburgers
Serve in a gluten free burger bun with lettuce and tomato.

Day 9
Breakfast
Citrus and Almond Salad with Ginger, Yoghurt and Blueberries
Ingredients
1 Valencia orange, peeled and segmented
2 mandarins, peeled and segmented
1 pink grapefruit, peeled and segmented
½ cup of dried cranberries
½ cup of blueberries
¼ teaspoon of cinnamon
1 tablespoons of honey
1 ½ cups of natural Greek yoghurt
½ cup of sliced almonds
Method
1. Place the orange, grapefruit and mandarin segments in a bowl cut them into halves (cut the grapefruit segments into thirds) and transfer the cut segments and any juice into a serving bowl.
2. Add the blueberries, cranberries honey and cinnamon, mix well and refrigerate for at least an hour.

Serving your Citrus and Almond Salad with Ginger, Yoghurt and Blueberries
Serve refrigerated with 2 tablespoons of Greek yoghurt.

Lunch
Quinoa Salad
Ingredients
1 cup of quinoa
1 white onion, finely chopped
2 carrots, roughly chopped
2 parsnips, roughly chopped
1 teaspoon thyme
Tahini dressing
Salt and ground black pepper
Olive oil
Method
- Coat the carrots, parsnips, and onion with a little olive oil and sprinkle over the thyme.
- Place the carrots, parsnips, and onion on a parchment lined baking tray and into a pre-heated oven at 425°F/200°C (gas mark 7), cook for 25-30 minutes turning midway.
- Whilst the vegetables roast cook the quinoa as per the instructions on the pack.
- Once cooked add the roasted vegetables to the quinoa and mix well.

Serving your Quinoa Salad
Serve hot with a dollop of tahini dressing.

Dinner
Salmon with Chili and Ginger
Ingredients
4-6 salmon fillets
2 cloves of garlic finely chopped
1 inch piece of ginger, grated
1 handful of fresh basil leaves, chopped
1 shallot, chopped
2 tablespoons of lemon juice
Salt and ground black pepper to taste
1 tablespoon of olive oil
1 tablespoon of butter
200g Asparagus
Green leaves
Method
1. In a large bowl mix together the garlic, ginger, basil leaves, shallot, lemon juice, olive oil and a little salt and pepper to taste.
2. Place the salmon into the mix and fully coat in the marinade, cover, and place in the fridge for at least 30 minutes.
3. Toss the Asparagus into some boiling water and cook for 4 minutes.
4. Heat the butter in a pan on a medium heat and place the salmon fillets skin down into to pan and cook for 3 minutes.
5. Gently turn the salmon over and cook for a further 3 minutes or until opaque.

Serving your Salmon with Chili and Ginger
Serve hot alongside the asparagus and some
green leaves.

Day 10
Breakfast
Blueberry Smoothie
Ingredients
1 cup of blueberries
½ cup of raspberries
½ cup of sliced cucumber
½ cup of soy milk
½ cup of natural yoghurt
1 tablespoon of condensed milk
Method
1. Add all the ingredients to a food processor or blender and blend until smooth.

Serving your Blueberry Smoothie
Serve immediately in a tall glass. Add ice during the blending process if the smoothie needs thickening.

Lunch
Sesame Prawn Stir Fry
Ingredients
450g fresh prawns
2 cloves of garlic, grated
1 large white onion, chopped
1 squash, chopped
2 cups shitake mushrooms
1 red bell pepper, chopped
4 tablespoons liquid Aminos
2 teaspoons sesame oil
2 tablespoon hemp seeds
2 tablespoon honey
Olive oil
Method
1. Heat 1 tablespoon of olive oil in a frying pan or skillet over a medium-high heat.
2. Add the prawns to the frying pan and cook for 3 minutes turning midway. Remove the frying pan from the heat and put the prawns to one side.
3. Whilst the prawns cook whisk together the sesame oil, Aminos liquid, honey and hemp seeds.
4. Heat 1 tablespoon of olive oil in a wok or large frying pan over a medium heat.
5. Add the garlic and onions to the frying pan and cook for 2 minutes before throwing in

the rest of the vegetables and stir fry for 5
minutes.

6. Pour the sauce into the pan and cook for a
    further 2-3 minutes.

Serving your Sesame Prawn Stir Fry
Serve with quinoa or brown rice (optional).

Dinner
Root Veg Tagine
Ingredients
400ml vegetable stock
1 bunch of carrots, roughly chopped
1 cup of kale
2 sweet potatoes, roughly chopped
2 parsnips, roughly chopped
1 large leek, roughly chopped
1 large red onion, chopped
½ teaspoon coriander
½ teaspoon cumin
½ teaspoon cinnamon
¼ teaspoon cayenne pepper
2 cloves of garlic, finely chopped
1 inch piece of ginger, grated or minced
2 tablespoons tomato puree
1 tablespoon lemon juice
Salt and ground black pepper
Olive oil
¼ cup chopped almonds
Method
1. Heat some olive oil in a large saucepan over a medium heat and cook the chopped onions for 2 minutes.

2. Add the parsnips to the saucepan and cook for 3 minutes before tossing in the almonds, cumin, coriander, cinnamon, cayenne, garlic, ginger, tomato puree and a little salt and pepper to taste.

3. Pour the vegetable stock into the pan along with the rest of the vegetables, bring to the boil and simmer for 18 minutes or until vegetables begin to soften.

Serving your Root Veg Tagine
Serve garnished with chopped almonds and bulgur wheat or quinoa.

Day 11
Breakfast
Toddy
Ingredients
250ml of soy or almond milk
¼ teaspoon of freshly grated ginger
¼ teaspoon cardamom
¼ teaspoon or turmeric
¼ teaspoon cinnamon
1 star anise
½ teaspoon of Manuka honey
A few drops of vanilla essence
Ground black pepper to taste
Method
1. In a saucepan, warm the soy or almond milk over a low to medium heat for 2-3 minutes.
2. Stir in all of the other ingredients and warm on a low heat for a further 2 minutes.
3. Pour the mixture through a fine sieve.

Serving
Serve warm.

Lunch
Mixed Peppers and Spinach Frittatas
Ingredients
100g spinach leaves
1 red bell pepper, diced
1 yellow bell pepper, diced
1 onion, chopped
6 large eggs
1 ½ teaspoons garam masala
Salt and ground black pepper to taste
½ cup of cheddar cheese
Method
1. Heat some oil in a large frying pan over a medium heat.
2. Throw the onions into the frying pan and sweat for 3 minutes or until soft.
3. Add the chopped peppers to the frying pan and cook for a further 3-5 minutes.
4. Mix the eggs and cheese and a little salt and ground black pepper to taste in a large mixing bowl or jug. When thoroughly mixed pour the mix onto the eggs and cook for 3 minutes
5. Top with an extra sprinkling of cheese and place the frying pan under the grill and cook for a further 5 minutes or until the frittata begins to brown.

Serving your Mixed Peppers and Spinach Frittatas

Cut into quarters and serve with a mixed green
leaf salad.

Dinner
Salmon Burgers
Ingredients
2 large salmon fillets
2 eggs, beaten
3 clove garlic, grated or minced
1 inch piece ginger, grated or minced
1 teaspoon cumin
½ teaspoon turmeric
¼ cup chopped walnuts
1 tablespoon multi-purpose (gluten free) flour
1 shallot, finely chopped
Salt and ground black pepper to taste
Olive oil
Method
1. Steam the salmon by wrapping it in tin foil and placing it in a pre-heated oven at 325°F/163°C (gas mark 3) for 8-10 minutes.
2. Remove the salmon from the oven and allow it to cool before placing the fillets into a large mixing bowl and breaking them apart using a fork.
3. Add the eggs, garlic, ginger, cumin, turmeric, walnuts, flour, shallots, and a little salt and pepper to taste to the bowl and mix well.
4. When mixed, use your hands to form the mix into 4-6 burger shapes.
5. Heat 1 tablespoon of olive oil in a frying pan or skillet over a medium heat.

6. Place the salmon burgers into the frying pan
    and cook for 5 minute turning midway.

Serving your Salmon Burgers
Serve with mayonnaise or a squeeze of lemon
juice and gluten free bread rolls.

Day 12
Breakfast
Orange and Carrot Detox + Cleanse
Ingredients
2 Valencia oranges peeled and segmented
12 carrots
2 beets
1 cup of Kale
4 sticks of celery
1 cucumber
2 cups of lettuce leaves
1 lemon
1 cup of spinach
1 teaspoon of grated ginger
½ cup fresh coriander
½ cup of ice
Method
1. Blend or juice all of the ingredients

Serving your Orange and Carrot Detox + Cleanse
Serve immediately.

Lunch
Salmon Chowder
Ingredients
1 large salmon fillet
¼ cup chopped carrot
¼ cup chopped celery
1 cup instant mash potato flakes
2 tablespoons chives, finely chopped
800ml chicken broth
2 cup cauliflower
¼ cup chopped dill
1 teaspoon dried tarragon
1 teaspoon mustard
Salt and ground black pepper to taste
Olive oil
Method
1. Heat some olive oil in a large saucepan over a medium heat.
2. Throw the carrot and the celery into the pan and cook for 3 minutes before adding the chicken stock and bringing to the boil.
3. Add the cauliflower, water, chives, and salmon and bring to the simmer for 8 minutes.
4. Remove the salmon fillet and break it apart using a fork before returning it to the mix along with the instant potato flakes, dill, tarragon, mustard and a little salt and pepper.

5. Cook on a low heat for 3-5 minutes, storing throughout.

Serving your Salmon Chowder
Serve hot with a side salad.

Dinner
Garlic and Mushroom Steak (see recipe above).

Day 13
Breakfast
Veggie Smoothie
Ingredients
2 cup spinach leaves
2 cups kale
5 carrots
2 tomatoes
½ cucumber, chopped
1 teaspoon grated ginger
¼ teaspoon turmeric
½ cup ice
Method
1. Blend or juice all of the ingredients.

Serving your Veggie Smoothie
Serve immediately.

Lunch
Zaatar Salmon with Citrus and Green leaf Salad (see recipe above).

Dinner
Spicy Chicken and Potato Curry
400g chicken, cubed
350g Maris Piper or Russet potatoes peeled and roughly cut into quarters
1 white onion chopped
3 cloves of garlic finely chopped
1 ½ inch piece of ginger, grated
1 ½ teaspoon garam masala
1 tin of chopped tomatoes
½ teaspoon medium heat chili powder
½ teaspoon cumin
¼ teaspoon coriander
½ teaspoon turmeric
1 tablespoon of olive oil
Salt and ground black pepper to taste
¼ cup of water
Method
1. Heat the olive oil in a large saucepan over a medium-high heat, when hot, throw in the onions, garlic, ginger and cook on a medium heat for 1-2 minutes.
2. Add chicken, garam masala, chili powder, cumin, coriander, turmeric and salt and pepper to taste and stir well.

3. Pour the tin of chopped tomatoes and water
    and add the potatoes into to saucepan, stir
    well.
4. Cook on a medium heat for 30-35 minutes or
    until the cooking liquids have reduced by half.

Serving your Spicy Chicken and Potato Curry
Serve hot with brown rice and gluten free
chapatti/roti.

Day 14
Breakfast
Blueberry Smoothie (see recipe above).
Lunch
Bacon and Cheese Frittatas
Ingredients
1 pack of smoked bacon, roughly chopped
1 cup of grated cheddar cheese
½ cup chopped spinach leaves
6 large eggs
Salt and black pepper to taste
Olive oil
Method
1. Heat some olive oil in a large frying pan and fry the bacon on a medium high heat for 3-4 minutes turning midway pour away and excess fats.
2. Whilst the bacon is cooking mix the eggs, cheese, spinach and a little salt and pepper to taste in a large mixing bowl.
3. Pour the eggs and cheese mixture over the bacon and cook for 3 minutes.
4. Top with an extra sprinkling of cheese and place the frying pan under the grill and cook for a further 5 minutes or until the frittata begins to brown.

Serving your Bacon and Cheese Frittatas
Serve hot with a green leaf salad.

Dinner
Salmon Burgers (see recipe above).

Day 15
Breakfast
Blueberry and Coconut Porridge
Ingredients
1 ½ cups of oats
3 cups of coconut milk
3 tablespoons of cocoa powder
¼ cup of blueberries
½ a banana sliced (optional)
Honey to taste
2 tablespoons coconut shavings
2 tablespoons of chia seeds
1 tablespoon of slivered almonds
Method
1. Place the oats, chia seeds, coconut milk, cocoa powder into a saucepan and simmer over a medium heat for 5 minutes or until the oats are cooked.
2. Mix in the honey and blueberries and pour into a serving bowl.

Serving your Blueberry and Coconut Porridge
Top the porridge with the banana slices, coconut shavings, slivered almonds and serve hot.

Lunch
Broccoli and Spinach Soup
Ingredients
5 cups of broccoli
5 cups of spinach
3 celery stalks, chopped
1 leek, chopped
800ml chicken stock
Salt and ground black pepper
¼ cup cheese of choice (parmesan is recommended)
Method
1. Heat some oil in a large saucepan.
2. Throw the leek in the pan and cook for 2-3 minutes before adding the stock and bring to the boil.
3. Add the broccoli and celery, cover and simmer for 5 minutes.
4. Remove the pan from the heat and add the spinach, cheese and a little salt and pepper to taste.
5. Blend until smooth using a food processor or blender.

Serving your Broccoli and Spinach Soup
Serve hot with gluten free bread rolls.

Dinner
Grilled Tandoori Chicken
Ingredients
500g boneless chicken, cubed.
1 teaspoon of garlic powder
1 teaspoon of ginger powder
2 teaspoons tandoori spice
½ teaspoon cumin
½ teaspoon turmeric
½ teaspoon fresh ground pepper
1 teaspoon medium-heat chili powder
Salt to taste
½ cup natural yoghurt
Method
1. Mix the spices together in a bowl along with the yoghurt.
2. Add the chicken, mix well ensure all the chicken is fully covered and refrigerate for at least 3 hours to overnight
3. Place the chicken under the grill and cook for 18-20 minutes, turning midway. The yoghurt will char but this is great for flavour.

Serving your Grilled Tandoori Chicken
Serve hot with baked potato, salad, and mayo.

Day 16
Breakfast
Blueberry and cinnamon (gluten-free)
Pancakes/Crepes
Ingredients
2 medium sized eggs
½ teaspoon of vanilla extract
¼ teaspoon of cinnamon
¼ teaspoon of sugar substitute (Splenda)
1 cup of gluten free multi-purpose flour
½ cup of almond or coconut or soy milk as preferred
½ cup of water
¼ teaspoon of salt
Coconut oil, 2 tablespoons of the pancake mix and ½ for the pan per pancake
¼ cup of blueberries
Honey
Method
1. Place 2 tablespoons of coconut oil in a frying pan on a medium heat.
2. In a large mixing bowl, whisk together the milk, vanilla extract, cinnamon, water, salt, sugar and eggs.
3. Slowly add the flour to the mix whisking throughout.
4. Pour the melted coconut oil into the mix and continue to whisk until the mix is fully combined.

5. Place ½ a tablespoon of coconut oil into the frying pan and warm over a medium heat.
6. Pour a small amount of the batter into the pan, around ½ a cup.
7. Whilst pouring the batter, be sure to tilt the pan ensuring the batter evenly covers the pan.
8. Cook the pancake over a medium-high heat for 1 ½ to 2 minutes or until golden.
9. Toss/flip the pancake and cook for a further 1-½ minutes or until golden.

Serving your Blueberry (gluten-free) Pancakes/Crepes
Lightly spread honey on the pancakes followed by some blueberries, roll them up and serve hot.

Lunch
Mediterranean Tuna Salad (see recipe above).

Dinner
Spicy Chicken and Potato Curry
400g chicken, cubed
350g Maris Piper or Russet potatoes peeled and roughly cut into quarters
1 white onion chopped
3 cloves of garlic finely chopped
1 ½ inch piece of ginger, grated
1 ½ teaspoon garam masala
1 tin of chopped tomatoes
½ teaspoon medium heat chili powder
½ teaspoon cumin
¼ teaspoon coriander
½ teaspoon turmeric
1 tablespoon of olive oil
Salt and ground black pepper to taste
¼ cup of water
Method

5. Heat the olive oil in a large saucepan over a medium-high heat, when hot, throw in the onions, garlic, ginger and cook on a medium heat for 1-2 minutes.

6. Add chicken, garam masala, chili powder, cumin, coriander, turmeric and salt and pepper to taste and stir well.

7. Pour the tin of chopped tomatoes and water and add the potatoes into to saucepan, stir well.

8. Cook on a medium heat for 30-35 minutes or
    until the cooking liquids have reduced by half.

Serving your Spicy Chicken and Potato Curry
Serve hot with rice and gluten free chapatti/roti

Day 17
Breakfast
Smoked Salmon and Potato Rosti (see recipe above).

Lunch
Simple Stuffed Mushrooms
Ingredients
4-6 portabella mushrooms washed with stalks removed and hollowed out
500g minced beef
1 green bell pepper, diced
1 red onion finely chopped
4 cloves of garlic finely chopped
1 ½ inch piece of ginger, grated
½ teaspoon cayenne pepper
½ teaspoon cumin
½ teaspoon turmeric
½ teaspoon paprika
1 teaspoon dried basil
Salt and ground black pepper
Olive oil
Cheese of choice, grated (optional)
Method
1. Heat some olive oil in a large saucepan over a medium-high heat.
2. Add the minced beef to the pan and cook for 4-6 minutes or until browning, pour away any excess fat.

3. Throw the onions into the pan, lower to a medium heat and cook for 2 minutes.

4. Dice the mushroom stalks and add them to the pan along with the rest of the peppers and all of the herbs and spices. Stir well and cook for 3 minutes.

5. Lightly process the beef and vegetable mix. The mixture should still appear roughly chopped, DO NOT process until smooth.

6. Take the beef and vegetable mix and stuff the portabella mushroom caps, do not overfill if you are adding cheese.

7. Top with grated cheese.

8. Place the mushroom on an oiled baking tray and into the oven on a medium heat for 18-20 minutes.

Serving your Simple Stuffed Mushrooms
Serve hot with steamed vegetables.

Dinner
Lemon and Herb Cod
Ingredients
2-4 cod loin fillets
1 small handful of chopped basil leaves
1 ½ teaspoons of Italian mixed herbs
¼ cup chopped parsley
1 tablespoon of lemon juice
1 tablespoon of lime juice
2 tablespoons of olive oil
Salt and ground black pepper to taste
Method
1. Mix together the basil, Italian mixed herbs, lemon juice, lime juice, chopped parsley, olive oil and a little salt and pepper to taste.
2. Coat the cod loins in the mix, cover and refrigerate for at least 30 minutes.
3. Heat some olive oil in a pan over a medium heat.
4. Place the cod loins into the pan, pour over any remaining marinade and cook for 4-6 minutes, turning midway.

Serving Lemon and Herb Cod
Serve with rice, spoon the juices from the pan over the cod and rice.

Day 18
Breakfast
Almond, Blueberry and Cinnamon Breakfast Bakes
Ingredients
¼ cup of slivered almonds
1 tablespoon of almond butter
2 cups of gluten free oats
¼ cup of dried blueberries
4 tablespoons of honey
1 teaspoon of chia seeds
1 ½ teaspoon of baking powder
1 teaspoon of ground cinnamon
½ teaspoon of vanilla extract
2 cups of coconut milk
A pinch of salt
Method
1. In a bowl, mix together the oats, baking powder and salt.
2. In a separate large bowl combine the honey, blueberries, chia seeds, cinnamon, coconut milk, vanilla extract and half of the slivered almonds.
3. Add the oats, baking powder and salt to the mix and stir thoroughly.
4. Preheat the oven to 370°F.
5. Lightly grease a baking tray with oil.
6. Evenly place the mix into the baking tray. Sprinkle on the remaining slivered almonds.

7. Bake for 25 minutes.

8. Lightly spread the almond butter on top of
    the bake and place back in the oven for a
    further 2-4 minutes.

9. Remove to the oven and place in a safe place
    to cool.

**Serving your Almond, Blueberry and
Cinnamon Breakfast Bakes**

These breakfast bakes are perfect for those with
little time, cook up a batch and eat this portable
breakfast treat throughout the week.

Lunch
Asparagus and Potato Frittata
Ingredients
125g asparagus tips
200g Maris Piper or King Edward potatoes
peeled and quartered
5 large eggs, beaten
1 onion, chopped
¼ cup of grated cheddar cheese
¼ teaspoon dried rosemary
¼ teaspoon dried thyme
Salt and ground black pepper to taste
Method
1. Boil some lightly salted water to the boil in a sauce pan, add the potatoes, bring to the simmer and cook for 6 minutes.
2. Add the asparagus tips to the saucepan and cook for a further 2-3 minutes.
3. Whilst the potatoes and asparagus cook, heat some oil in a large frying pan over a medium heat.
4. Throw the onions into the frying pan and sweat for 4-6 minutes or until soft.
5. Drain the asparagus and potatoes and put them to one side.
6. Mix the eggs, thyme, rosemary, and cheese in a large mixing bowl or jug, when thoroughly mixed pour the mix onto the eggs.

7. Haphazardly add the asparagus and potatoes to the frying pan with the eggs, cheese, and onions, cook for 5-8 minutes.

8. Top with an extra sprinkling of cheese and place the frying pan under the grill and cook for a further 5-7 minutes or until the frittata begins to brown.

Serving your Asparagus and Potato Frittata
Cut into quarters and serve.

Dinner
Simple Stuffed Mushrooms
Ingredients
4-6 portabella mushrooms washed with stalks
removed and hollowed out
500g minced beef
1 green bell pepper, diced
1 red onion finely chopped
4 cloves of garlic finely chopped
1 ½ inch piece of ginger, grated
½ teaspoon cayenne pepper
½ teaspoon cumin
½ teaspoon turmeric
½ teaspoon paprika
1 teaspoon dried basil
Salt and ground black pepper
Olive oil
Cheese of choice, grated (optional)
Method

9. Heat some olive oil in a large saucepan over a medium-high heat.

10. Add the minced beef to the pan and cook for 4-6 minutes or until browning, pour away any excess fat.

11. Throw the onions into the pan, lower to a medium heat and cook for 2 minutes.

12. Dice the mushroom stalks and add them to the pan along with the rest of the peppers

and all of the herbs and spices. Stir well and cook for 3 minutes.

13. Lightly process the beef and vegetable mix. The mixture should still appear roughly chopped, DO NOT process until smooth.
14. Take the beef and vegetable mix and stuff the portabella mushroom caps, do not overfill if you are adding cheese.
15. Top with grated cheese.
16. Place the mushroom on an oiled baking tray and into the oven on a medium heat for 18-20 minutes.

Serving your Simple Stuffed Mushrooms
Serve hot with steamed vegetables.

Day 19
Breakfast
Blueberry and Coconut Porridge
Ingredients
1 ½ cups of oats
3 cups of coconut milk
3 tablespoons cocoa powder
¼ cup of blueberries
½ cup of raspberries
½ teaspoon Manuka honey
2 tablespoons of coconut shavings
2 tablespoons of chia seeds
1 tablespoon of slivered almonds
Method

3. Place the oats, chia seeds, coconut milk, cocoa powder into a saucepan and simmer over a medium heat for 5 minutes or until the oats are cooked.
4. Mix in the honey, blueberries and pour into a serving bowl.

Serving your Blueberry and Coconut Porridge
Top the porridge with coconut shavings and slivered almonds, serve hot.

Lunch
5 Minute Salad (see recipe above).

Dinner
Mediterranean Stuffed Peppers
Ingredients
4 red bell peppers
½ cup chopped red onion
2 cloves of garlic finely chopped
1 inch fresh ginger, grated
2 teaspoons Italian mixed spice
½ handful chopped fresh basil leaves
1 cup fresh spinach, chopped
1 courgette, diced
3 red chili, finely chopped
1 cup chopped mushrooms
1 cup quinoa
½ cup passata
1 tablespoon of tomato puree
Salt and ground black pepper to taste
Olive oil
Cheeses of choice (optional)
Method
1. Cook the quinoa as per the instructions on the packet; this tends to be for between 12-15 minutes.
2. Warm some olive oil in a pan over a medium heat.
3. Throw in onions into the pan along with the garlic and ginger and cook for 2 minutes.
4. Add the mushrooms, courgette, spinach, Italian mixed herbs, basil, chili and a little salt

and ground black pepper to taste and cook for 1-2 minutes.

5. Stir the passata and tomato puree into the vegetable mix and cook on a medium-low heat for 3-5 minutes.

6. Whilst the vegetables and quinoa cook wash the bell peppers, cut off the tops and remove all the seeds and stem.

7. When cooked add the quinoa to the vegetables and mix thoroughly.

8. Stuff the empty peppers with the vegetable and quinoa mix, and top with grated cheese (optional)

9.   Lightly spray with olive oil, place on a baking tray and cook at 400°F/200°C (gas mark 5) for 25-35 minutes.

Serving your Mediterranean Stuffed Peppers
Allow 3 minutes to slightly cool and serve.

Day 20
Breakfast
Honey and Pineapple anti-inflammatory special
Ingredients
Half a pineapple
1 lime
1 teaspoon grated ginger
2 carrots
1 tablespoon of Manuka honey
½ cup Greek yoghurt
½ cup of ice
Method
1. Blend together or juice the pineapple, lime, carrots, honey, yoghurt and ginger.

Serving your Honey and Pineapple anti-inflammatory special
Serve immediately.

Lunch
The Ultimate Veggie Burger (see recipe above).

Dinner
Grilled Tandoori Chicken (see recipe above).

Day 21
Breakfast
Smoked Salmon and Runny Egg on Toast (see recipe above).

Lunch
Mixed Peppers and Spinach Frittatas (see recipe above).

Dinner
Salmon with Chili and Ginger
Ingredients
4-6 salmon fillets
2 cloves of garlic finely chopped
1 inch piece of ginger, grated
1 handful of fresh basil leaves, chopped
1 shallot, chopped
2 tablespoons of lemon juice
Salt and ground black pepper to taste
1 tablespoon of olive oil
1 tablespoon of butter
200g Asparagus
Green leaves
Method
6. In a large bowl mix together the garlic, ginger, basil leaves, shallot, lemon juice, olive oil and a little salt and pepper to taste.
7. Place the salmon into the mix and fully coat in the marinade, cover, and place in the fridge for at least 30 minutes.

8. Toss the Asparagus into some boiling water
    and cook for 4 minutes.
9. Heat the butter in a pan on a medium heat
    and place the salmon fillets skin down into to
    pan and cook for 3 minutes.
10. Gently turn the salmon over and cook for a
    further 3 minutes or until opaque.

Serving your Salmon with Chili and Ginger
Serve hot alongside the asparagus and some
green leaves.

Day 22
Breakfast
**Cucumber, Ginger and Pineapple Breakfast
Smoothie (see recipe above)**

Lunch
Lentil Soup
Ingredients
2 cups of lentils
800ml chicken stock
2 cloves of garlic finely chopped
3 carrots, peeled and chopped
1 cup of chopped celery
1 white onion finely chopped
1 tablespoon or lemon juice
½ teaspoon of paprika
½ teaspoon of cumin
1 teaspoon of ground black pepper
¼ teaspoon of salt
Method
1. Warm some olive oil in a saucepan and throw in the garlic, carrots, onion, celery, salt and pepper.
2. Cook on a medium heat for 5 minutes.
3. Pour the chicken stock, lentils, lemon juice, paprika, cumin into the saucepan and stir well, bring to the simmer and cook for 18-20 minutes.
4. Blend and serve.

Serving you Lentil Soup
Serve hot with a gluten free bread roll.

Dinner
Ginger Beef and Broccoli Stir-Fry (see recipe above).

Day 23
Breakfast
Almond, Blueberry and Cinnamon Breakfast Bakes (see recipe above).

Lunch
Spicy Carrot and Tomato Soup
Ingredients
2 large tomatoes, chopped
1 packet of sun-dried tomatoes, chopped
2 Large carrots peeled and chopped
1 red chili pepper, chopped
1 large onion, chopped
3 sticks of celery
2 cloves of garlic finely chopped
1 teaspoon of dried cumin
1 tablespoon of tomato puree
1 teaspoon medium heat chili powder
½ teaspoon paprika
Salt and ground black pepper to taste
800ml chicken stock
Olive oil
Method
1. Heat a little olive oil in a saucepan over a medium heat and throw in the onion, garlic and cook for 2 minutes stirring throughout
2. Mix in the chicken stock, tomatoes, carrots, chili pepper, celery, cumin, tomato puree, chili powder, paprika and a little salt and ground black pepper to taste.

3. Simmer for 18 minutes.
4. Blend until smooth using a food processor,
    return to a low heat and cook for 3-5
    minutes.

Serving your Spicy Carrot and Tomato Soup
Serve hot with a gluten free bread roll.

Dinner
Tomato and Herb Sea bass
Ingredients
2-4 sea bass fillets
1 packet of sun-dried tomatoes, chopped
1 handful of cherry tomatoes, chopped
½ teaspoon of dried basil
1 teaspoon of mixed herbs
2 tablespoon tomato puree
2 cloves of garlic finely chopped
½ white onion, finely chopped
Salt and ground black pepper to taste
150g spinach leaves
Method
1. Mix the sun-dried tomatoes, cherry tomatoes and crush them with the back of a spoon.
2. Add the mixed herbs, basil, tomato puree, garlic, onions, salt and ground black pepper.
3. Coat the sea bass in the tomato and herb marinade, cover and refrigerate for at least 2 hours.
4. Preheat the oven to 400°F/200°C (gas mark 6).
5. Place the sea bass in a ceramic dish along with the marinade sauce and cook for 15 minutes.

Serving your Tomato and Herb Sea bass
Serve hot atop a bed of fresh spinach leaves.

Day 24
Breakfast
Cinnamon and Oatmeal Gingerbreads
Ingredients
1 cup of coarse oatmeal
1 teaspoon of cinnamon
¼ teaspoon of cloves
¼ teaspoon of ginger
¼ teaspoon of cardamom
¼ teaspoon of allspice
1 tablespoon of honey
Water as specified by coarse oatmeal packet cooking instructions
Method
1. Cook the coarse oatmeal as specified on its packaging and mix in all of the spices whilst cooking.
2. Once the coarse oatmeal is cooked, mix in the honey and leave to cool.

Serving your Cinnamon and Oatmeal Gingerbreads
Just snap off a piece of this breakfast treat and be on your way. Ideal for travel and lasts at least 3 days if properly stored.

Lunch
Spicy Chicken and Potato Curry
400g chicken, cubed
350g Maris Piper or Russet potatoes peeled and roughly cut into quarters
1 white onion chopped
3 cloves of garlic finely chopped
1 ½ inch piece of ginger, grated
1 ½ teaspoon garam masala
1 tin of chopped tomatoes
½ teaspoon medium heat chili powder
½ teaspoon cumin
¼ teaspoon coriander
½ teaspoon turmeric
1 tablespoon of olive oil
Salt and ground black pepper to taste
¼ cup of water
Method
1. Heat the olive oil in a large saucepan over a medium-high heat, when hot, throw in the onions, garlic, ginger and cook on a medium heat for 1-2 minutes.

2. Add chicken, garam masala, chili powder, cumin, coriander, turmeric and salt and pepper to taste and stir well.

3. Pour the tin of chopped tomatoes and water and add the potatoes into to saucepan, stir well.

4. Cook on a medium heat for 30-35 minutes or
    until the cooking liquids have reduced by half.

Serving your Spicy Chicken and Potato Curry
Serve hot with rice and gluten free chapatti/roti.

Dinner
Mediterranean Stuffed Peppers (see recipe above)

Day 25
Breakfast
Poached Egg on Toast
Ingredients
2 large eggs
Brown bread (gluten free)
¼ teaspoon of vinegar
Method

- Bring a pan of water to the simmer over a medium heat and add the vinegar.
- Crack the eggs into ramekins, 1 egg per ramekin.
- Using a spoon, create a whirlpool in the simmering water, this will help the egg whites to surround and wrap the yolks.
- Carefully tip the eggs into the water whites first.
- Cook for 3 minutes.
- Whilst the eggs cook toast the bread in a toaster or under the grill.
- Remove the poached eggs from the water using a slotted spoon cutting off any uneven and wispy edges.
- Drain off any excess poaching water from the eggs.

Serving your Poached Egg on Toast
Top each piece of toast with a poached egg and serve.

Lunch
Asparagus and Potato Frittata (see recipe above).

Dinner
Pan Seared Salmon and Mushrooms
Ingredients
2-4 skinless/deboned salmon fillets
1 cup sliced shitake mushrooms
½ tablespoon lemon juice
½ tablespoon lime juice
½ teaspoon medium-heat chili flakes
1 tablespoon black pepper
Salt to taste
½ tablespoon chopped chives
½ tablespoon parsley
Olive oil
Method
1. Heat 1 tablespoon of olive oil in a large frying pan or skillet on a medium heat.
2. Add the mushrooms to the pan along with the chili flakes and cook for 3 minutes.
3. Coat the top side of the salmon with black pepper, place into the frying pan and cook for 3 minutes before carefully turning and cooking for a further 2 minutes.
4. Remove the salmon from the frying pan and pour over the lemon and lime juices.

Serving your Pan Seared Salmon and Mushrooms

Garnish with chives and parsley, serve hot with brown rice or quinoa.

Day 26
Breakfast
Blueberry and Coconut Porridge (see recipe above).

Lunch
Beetroot Salad (see recipe above).

Dinner
Dry Rub Chicken
Ingredients
500g boneless chicken, cubed.
1 teaspoon of garlic powder
1 teaspoon of ginger powder
1 teaspoon mustard powder
½ Teaspoon cumin
½ teaspoon turmeric
½ teaspoon fresh ground pepper
Salt to taste
Method
1. Mix the spices together in a bowl.
2. Generously apply an even coating of the dry rub mix to the chicken and refrigerate for at least 2 hours.
3. Place the chicken under the grill and cook for 16-20 minutes or until charred, turning midway.

Serving your Dry Rub Chicken
Serve hot with baked potato, salad, and mayo

Day 27
Breakfast
Green Detox Smoothie (see recipe above).

Lunch
Citrus, Avocado and Green Leaf Salad (see recipe above).

Dinner
Lemon and Herb Cod
Ingredients
2-4 cod loin fillets
1 small handful of chopped basil leaves
1 ½ teaspoons of Italian mixed herbs
¼ cup chopped parsley
1 tablespoon of lemon juice
1 tablespoon of lime juice
2 tablespoons of olive oil
Salt and ground black pepper to taste
Method
1. Mix together the basil, Italian mixed herbs, lemon juice, lime juice, chopped parsley, olive oil and a little salt and pepper to taste.
2. Coat the cod loins in the mix, cover and refrigerate for at least 30 minutes.
3. Heat some olive oil in a pan over a medium heat.
4. Place the cod loins into the pan, pour over any remaining marinade and cook for 4-6 minutes, turning midway.

Serving Lemon and Herb Cod
Serve with rice, spoon the juices from the pan
over the cod and rice.

Day 28
Breakfast
Salmon and Avocado on Toast

Lunch
Asparagus and Potato Frittata (see recipe above)

Dinner
Bulgur Stuffed Mushrooms
4-6 portabella mushrooms washed with stalks removed and hollowed out
1 cup bulgur wheat
800ml chicken stock
200ml chicken stock
1 red bell pepper, diced
1 red onion finely chopped
4 cloves of garlic finely chopped
1 ½ inch piece of ginger, grated
½ teaspoon cayenne pepper
½ teaspoon cumin
½ teaspoon turmeric
½ teaspoon paprika
1 teaspoon dried basil
Salt and ground black pepper
1 teaspoon of sugar
1 packet of dried apricots, finely chopped
Olive oil
Method
1. Cook the bulgur wheat as instructed by the packet.

2. Heat some olive oil in a large pan on a
   medium heat.
3. Throw the onions into the pan, lower to a
   medium heat and cook for 2 minutes.
4. Dice the mushroom stalks and add them to
   the pan along with the rest of the peppers
   and all of the herbs and spices. Stir well and
   cook for 3 minutes.
5. When the bulgur wheat is cooked mix it with
   the vegetable mix and gently stuff the
   mushroom caps with the mix.
6. Cook in the oven on a medium heat for 15-
   18minutes.
7. In a small sauce pan pour the200ml chicken
   stock along with the dried apricots and sugar
   and place on a medium-low heat.
8. Gently crush the apricots with the back of a
   spoon whilst cooking, stir throughout, until
   the liquids have reduced by half.

Serving your Bulgur stuffed Mushrooms
Serve hot with steamed kale or fresh green leaf
salad.

Snacks (secret bonus chapter)

Greek Yoghurt with Almonds Berries and Granola

Ingredients

1 medium sized pot of Greek yoghurt

½ cup blueberries

¼ cup raspberries

¼ cup of crushed almonds

¼ crushed walnuts

2 tablespoons chia seeds

¼ cup granola of choice

Method

1. Toss all of the ingredients in a bowl and mix thoroughly.

2. Separate into 4-6 ramekins and refrigerate.

Serving your Greek Yoghurt with Almonds Berries and Granola

Serve chilled.

Cinnamon Baked Apples
Ingredients
4-6 apples, cored but not peeled
½ teaspoon of nutmeg
1 teaspoon of cinnamon
¼ teaspoon of dried cloves
¼ cup of mixed nuts, crushed
2 tablespoons of honey
½ piece ginger, grated
¼ cup of dried cranberries
1 cup of apple juice (not from concentrate)
Method
1. Mix the nutmeg, cinnamon, cloves, mixed nuts, ginger and cranberries in a bowl.
2. Stuff the apple with the mix, place on a parchment lined baking tray and evenly pour the honey over them.
3. Pour the apple juice around the apple to stop them drying out whilst being cooked.
4. Place the apples in a pre-heated oven at 325°F/160°C (gas mark 3) for 30 minutes.
5. Allow to cool slightly before serving.

Serving you Cinnamon Baked Apples
Serve warm with (dairy free) ice cream.

Cumin Roasted Carrots
Ingredients
350g carrots, chopped julienne
1 teaspoon of Cumin
Salt and ground black pepper to taste
1 tablespoon olive oil
Method
1. Mix the cumin and olive oil with a little salt and ground pepper, generously coat the carrots and refrigerate for at least 30 minutes.
2. Preheat the oven to 400°F/200°C (gas mark 6) and cook the carrots for 26-28 minutes.

Serving your Cumin Roasted Carrots
Serve hot with salmon or simply eat as a delicious and healthy snack.

Garlic Roasted Potato Hash
Ingredients
500g Maris Piper potatoes, peeled, sliced and cubed
2 cloves of garlic finely chopped
1 teaspoon of dried rosemary
2 tablespoons of olive oil
Salt and ground black pepper to taste
Method
1. Mix the garlic, dried rosemary, olive oil and salt and black pepper to taste.
2. Coat the potato cubes in the marinade mix and place into a pre-heated oven.
3. Cook the potatoes and any remaining marinade at 400/200°C (gas mark 6) for 25 minutes.

Serving your Garlic Roasted Potato Hash
Serve hot, an ideal side fish and salad dishes.

Garlic Roasted Broccoli
Ingredients
3 cups of broccoli florets
3 cloves of garlic finely chopped
2 teaspoons of butter
Salt and Ground Pepper to taste
Olive oil
Method
1. Preheat the oven to 425°F/210°C (gas mark 6).
2. Mix together the butter, olive oil, garlic and a little salt and ground pepper in a bowl.
3. Place the broccoli on a baking tray and evenly pour over the oil mix.
4. Cook for 20 minutes (or until stems are crisp and tender) turning midway.

Serving your Garlic Roasted Broccoli
Serve hot.

Fried Okra
Ingredients
400g okra, sliced into strips
½ cup all-purpose gluten free flour
1 teaspoon paprika
1 teaspoon cayenne pepper
2 cloves of garlic finely chopped
Salt and ground black pepper
¼ cup of water
1 cup of olive oil
Method
1. Mix the flour, paprika, garlic, cayenne and a little salt and ground black pepper in a bowl and slowly add the water stirring/whisking continuously.
2. Pour the olive oil into a saucepan and warm over a medium-high heat.
3. Coat the okra slices in the seasoned batter mix ensuring they are all fully and evenly covered.
4. Fry the Okra for 4-5 minutes or they appear to darken and crisp.

Serving your Fried Okra
Serve hot with sour cream dip as the perfect snack or side.

Cauliflower Cheese
Ingredients
3 cups of cauliflower
400ml milk
1 ½ cups of grated cheddar cheese
1 tablespoon of butter
1 tablespoon of flour
Salt and ground black pepper
Method

1. Season the cauliflower with some salt and ground black pepper to taste.
2. Boil some water in a saucepan.
3. Toss in the cauliflower and simmer for 5-7 minutes.
4. Before the cauliflower is ready, melt the butter in a saucepan over a medium heat.
5. Add the milk to the butter and stir until the milk begins to simmer.
6. Lower the heat and begin to add and stir in the grated cheddar a little at a time until melted.
7. If the cheese sauce still seems a little watery, add flour and stir until the sauce begins to thicken, add Salt and ground black pepper to taste.
8. Remove the cauliflower from the saucepan and pat dry using kitchen towel.

Serving your Cauliflower Cheese

Serve hot with a generous pouring of the cheese
sauce.

Garlic Hummus
Ingredients
3 cloves of garlic
500g chickpeas
¼ cup of chives
1 teaspoon salt
3 tablespoons of water
¼ teaspoon cayenne pepper
2 tablespoons sesame tahini
Olive oil
Method
1. Place the garlic on foil, pour 1 teaspoon of olive oil over the garlic and seal by folding the foil over.
2. Roast the garlic in a pre-heated oven at 400°F/200°C (gas mark 6) for 20 minutes.
3. Remove the garlic from the oven when soft and place into a food processor or blender along with the chickpeas, chives, cayenne, salt, tahini, water and 1 tablespoon of olive oil.

Serving your Garlic Hummus
Serve with gluten free bread sticks.

Kale Crisps
Ingredients
1 large packet of kale
1 cup of grated sweet potato
1 cup cashews, soaked for 2 hours
1 lemon, juiced
1 tablespoon honey
2 tablespoons fresh water
Salt to taste
Method
1. Blend together the sweet potato, cashews, honey, lemon juice, water and a little salt to taste using a food processor or blender until smooth.
2. Place the kale in a large mixing bowl and, the paste from the blender and mix well ensuring all the kale is evenly covered.
3. Place the kale on a parchment lined baking tray and cook on 150°F/70°C (gas mark 1) for 2 hours or until fully dehydrated.
4. Allow the kale crisps to cool before serving.

Serving your Kale Crisps
Serve anytime. Kale crisps can be stored for up to a week.

Afterword

You did it, congratulations!

I really hope that you enjoyed **Reverse Diabetes: Proven Methods for Safely Lowering Blood Sugar and Reversing Diabetes without Drugs, Including Free 28 Day Recipe Plan** and that it supports you alongside your doctor and medical team in taking action, tackling and taking back control of your diabetic diagnosis. By now you should be enjoying the sense of accomplishment that comes with a clean and healthy lifestyle and soon it will infect of every aspect of your life. Through focussing on working on one aspect of our lives at a time, we have the ability to leverage our accomplishments against one another in order to gain greater power and freedom over diabetes. When we do this we will see our lives transformed, we will feel more stable, and relaxed, which as we now know, will serve to lower our blood pressure!

I wish you all the bet of health

Evelyn Halliday

www.ingramcontent.com/pod-product-compliance
Lightning Source LLC
Chambersburg PA
CBHW051100250726
48656CB00001B/402